Copyright 2023

Table of Contents

Cerebrovascular Disease

Cerebrovascular disease is a term for conditions that affect blood flow to your brain. Conditions include stroke, brain aneurysm, brain bleed and carotid artery disease. These conditions are medical emergencies and need prompt treatment, such as medications and surgery. Though disability or death may occur, some people make a full recovery.

BREAKFAST

1. Apple Strudel

Prep Time: 10 Minutes

Cook Time: 35 Minutes

Servings: 6

Ingredients

- 1 sheet of vegan frozen puff pastry thawed (gluten-free if needed)
- 4 medium (500 g) diced apples peeled and cored
- 1 squeeze of lemon juice
- 1/2 scant cup (50 g) walnuts chopped
- 1/3 cup (50 g) raisins (see notes)
- 1/4 cup (50 g) sugar of choice + more for sprinkling on top (see notes)
- 1/4 tsp. vanilla bean paste or 1/2 tsp. vanilla extract
- 1 heaped Tbsp. cinnamon
- 1 Pinch of ground ginger
- 1 Pinch of cardamom

Instructions

1. First, preheat the oven to 350 °F/180 °C and roll out the sheet of puff pastry, placing it on a baking tray. I use the parchment paper it comes with to line the baking sheet.

2. Then, rinse and chop the apples into ½-inch pieces and transfer them to a large bowl with the remaining filling ingredients. Stir well.

3. Pour the apple mixture over the strudel dough, forming a rectangular mound in the middle with a 2-inch border all the way around.

4. To seal the apple strudel, first, fold the top and bottom up and over the filling. Then, carefully fold in both sides, pinching at the seams to seal it.

5. If there are a few small cracks, that's fine. However, if you want to try to fix them, use a damp finger and gently smooth/pinch them closed.

6. (OPTIONAL STEP) For a more browned top, brush the pastry with melted vegan butter and sprinkle it with coarse sugar of choice.

7. Transfer the apple strudel to the oven, seam side down, and bake for about 35 minutes until lightly golden brown on the outside.

8. Allow it to cool on a wire rack for 10 minutes, then dust with powdered sugar (or powdered Erythritol), slice, and serve!

9. My favorite way to serve this dessert is with a scoop of vegan vanilla ice cream, warm vegan custard/ vanilla sauce, or dairy-free whipped cream.

Prep Time: 10 Minutes

Cook Time: 10 Minutes

Servings: 7

Ingredients

- 1 Oz (28 g) dried mushrooms or use 200 g fresh
- 2 3/4 cups (650 ml) low-sodium vegetable broth
- 1 Tbsp oil or water
- 1 onion diced
- 3 cloves of garlic minced
- 4 Tbsp (32 g) cornstarch (or arrowroot flour)
- Salt and black pepper to taste
- 1/3 cup (80 ml) dairy-free milk of choice
- 1 Tbsp tamari or soy sauce
- 1/4 cup (60 ml) red wine (optional)
- 3/4 tsp fresh thyme
- 1 1/2 tsp fresh rosemary

Instructions

1. You can the in the post for visual instructions.
2. Add the dried mushrooms to a large pot or saucepan with the vegetable broth, bring it to a boil, allow it to cook for about 1 minute before turning off the heat and setting it aside. Meanwhile, finely dice the onion and mince the garlic and fresh herbs.

3. If you're using fresh mushrooms, sauté them in a skillet to remove excess liquid, and they begin to brown (don't overcrowd the pan).
4. Heat the oil in a large skillet over medium heat. Once hot, add the onion and sauté for 2-3 minutes. Then, add the garlic, herbs, and seasonings, and sauté for another minute, stirring frequently.
5. Meanwhile, in a small bowl, combine the plant-based milk and cornstarch and stir/whisk until lump-free.
6. Next, deglaze the skillet with the soy sauce and red wine (optional) while stirring to scrape up any bits from the bottom of the pan.
7. Pour in the mushroom and broth mixture and stir to combine. Then stir in the cornstarch milk mixture and let the gravy simmer and thicken for about 5 minutes.
8. The longer you leave it to simmer, the thicker and more flavorful the vegan mushroom sauce/ gravy will become.
9. Then, either use an immersion blender directly in the pot or transfer it to a stand blender and blend until smooth.
10. If the gravy is too thick, add more vegetable broth. If it's too thin, add more cornstarch (in a slurry) and heat on the stovetop until thickened, stirring constantly.
11. Finally, taste and adjust any of the seasonings and enjoy over mashed potatoes, vegan meatloaf, vegan meatballs, etc.

Prep Time: 15 Minutes

Cook Time: 5 Minutes

Servings: 8

Ingredients

- 1 cup (240 ml) dairy-free milk
- 1 roasted red pepper
- 2 Tbsp (15 g) agar powder (100% strength)
- 3/4-1 tsp salt
- 1 tsp onion powder
- 1 tsp garlic powder
- 1/2 tsp smoked paprika
- 1/8 tsp turmeric powder
- 4 Tbsp nutritional yeast (optional but recommended)
- 1/4 cup (60 g) tahini or cashew butter
- 1 Tbsp (25 g) tomato paste
- 1/3 cup (80 ml) olive brine
- 1 1/2 Tbsp tapioca flour

Instructions

1. Grease the inside of a small/medium bowl or container of choice (mine measures 5.5 x 3 inches / 14 x 7.5 cm) with a neutral oil and set aside.
2. Add all ingredients (except the olive brine and tapioca flour) to a blender and blend until completely smooth.
3. Transfer the mixture to a saucepan and bring it to a simmer over medium heat, stirring frequently. Once it

simmers, set your timer to 4 minutes. Let it simmer over low heat and stir occasionally as it gets pretty thick.

4. In a small bowl, mix the olive brine with tapioca flour. It's important that the juice is not cold (otherwise, it will make the cheese sauce set partially). Add the mixture to the saucepan and stir with a whisk.

5. Continue to simmer for 1 minute, it will thicken even more, so I recommend stirring frequently. Then immediately pour the cheese sauce into the prepared bowl (it hardens fast, so try to be quick) and press it down with a spatula.

6. Let it cool until the bowl is just slightly warm, not hot, then refrigerate for at least 2-3 hours (or overnight) until set. Enjoy with crackers!

Prep Time: 35 Minutes

Cook Time: 25 Minutes

Servings: 6

Ingredients

- 2 pounds (900 g) potatoes (e.g. Yukon Gold) peeled and sliced
- 3 cups (400 g) pumpkin chopped into 1-inch cubes
- 1 cup (200 g) dried lentils e.g. brown
- 2 cups (480 ml) vegetable broth or salted water
- 1 tbsp vegetable oil divided
- 1 large onion diced
- 3 cloves of garlic minced
- 1 batch of (200 g) vegan cheese sauce or 7 oz (200 g) vegan queso
- 2/3 cup (150 g) vegan cream cheese (or use cashew cream)
- 1/2 tbsp onion powder
- 1 tsp garlic powder
- 1 tsp ground cumin
- 1/2 tsp ground nutmeg
- 1/2 tsp smoked paprika
- 1/4 tsp red pepper flakes
- Salt & black pepper to taste
- Fresh herbs to garnish (e.g. parsley or thyme)
- Fried onion rings to garnish (optional)

Instructions

Prepare the Ingredients:

1. First, rinse the lentils well, removing any debris. Then soak them in lukewarm water for 15 minutes. Drain the water once done.
2. This step is optional, but helps to make the lentils more easily digestible, plus they cook faster.
3. Meanwhile, peel and slice the potatoes into 1/4-inch slices (6 mm). Then, transfer them to a large pot of salted water and cook until fork-tender (about 10 minutes), being careful not to overcook them.
4. While the potatoes cook, finely chop the onion and garlic, and chop the pumpkin into 1-inch cubes.
5. In a large saucepan, heat some oil, add the onion, and sauté over medium heat for 3-4 minutes. Add the garlic, spices, lentils, and broth and bring to a boil. Lower the heat to a simmer, and allow it to cook for about 15 minutes until no liquid remains in the pot.
6. ASSEMBLE
7. While the lentils cook, preheat the oven to 390 °F/200 °C, and prepare the vegan cheese sauce (if using). Then combine the vegan cream cheese (or cashew cream) and the cheese sauce (or store-bought vegan queso).
8. Sauté the pumpkin in a pan with a little oil for 3-5 minutes.
9. To assemble the potato bake, start by adding a layer of the cooked potatoes (about half of them) to a greased baking dish (around 9x13).
10. Then, add a layer of the lentils, followed by half the vegan cheese mixture.
11. Next, add the sautéed pumpkin, followed by the remaining potato slices.

12. Finally, pour over the remaining vegan cheese mixture and bake the vegetable potato bake in the oven for 25 minutes.
13. Allow it to cool for a few minutes, garnish with fried onions (if using) and fresh herbs, and enjoy!

Prep Time: 15 Minutes

Cook Time: 40 Minutes

Servings: 9

Ingredients

Dry Cake Ingredients:

- 1 cup (90 g) oat flour (gluten-free if needed)
- 1/2 cup (80 g) rice flour
- 2 Tbsp (16 g) cornstarch or potato starch
- 1/3 cup (70 g) Erythritol or sugar
- 1 1/2 tsp baking powder
- 1/4 tsp baking soda
- 1/2 tsp sea salt

Wet Cake Ingredients:

- 3/4 cup (180 ml) almond milk or any other dairy-free milk
- 2/3 cup (160 g) applesauce unsweetened
- 2 Tbsp (28 g) oil
- 1 Tbsp apple cider vinegar
- 1 tsp vanilla extract

Streusel:

- 1/2 cup (80 g) rice flour or regular flour, if you're not gluten-free
- 1/2 cup (60 g) almond flour or shredded unsweetened coconut
- 1/4 cup (40 g) coconut sugar or brown sugar

- 2 Tbsp (28 g) oil
- 2 Tbsp (40 g) maple syrup or any other liquid sweetener
- 2 tsp cinnamon
- 1/4 tsp sea salt

Instructions

1. I recommend measuring the ingredients in grams on a kitchen scale. Check the video in the post for visual instructions.
2. Start by lining a baking dish with parchment paper with an overhang on all sides (for easy removal). My pan measures 6×9 inches (ca. 15x23 cm).
3. Make the streusel topping: Add all dry ingredients for the streusel to a bowl, stir with a whisk, then add the wet ingredients. Use your fingers to combine everything until the mixture is slightly crumbly. Set aside and preheat your oven to 350 degrees Fahrenheit (ca. 180 °C).
4. Add all dry cake ingredients into a large mixing bowl and stir with a whisk. You could also add the dry ingredients to a food processor and blend for a couple of seconds.
5. Next, add the wet cake ingredients and stir with a whisk. You can also use a hand mixer.
6. Assemble: Pour about half of the batter into the lined baking dish. Then add half of the cinnamon streusel. Pour the remaining batter on top of the streusel and finally add the remaining streusel.
7. Bake for about 35-40 minutes, or until a toothpick inserted into the center of the crumb cake comes out almost clean (it can be crumbly but shouldn't be wet).

The baking time can be a few minutes less or more, depending on your oven and the size of the pan. Let cool completely, then drizzle with icing (optional). Check the recipe notes below for the icing. Enjoy!

Prep Time: 5 Minutes

Cook Time: 35 Minutes

Servings: 8

Ingredients

Dry ingredients:

- 2 cups (180 g) quick oats (gluten-free if needed)
- 2 Tbsp ground chia seeds or flax seeds
- 2 tsp pumpkin spice
- 1 tsp ground cinnamon
- 1/4 tsp salt
- 1 tsp baking powder

Wet ingredients:

- 1 cup (240 g) pumpkin purée
- 3 Tbsp (50 g) nut/seed butter of choice
- 3 Tbsp (60 g) maple syrup or any other liquid sweetener
- 1 1/2 tsp vanilla extract
- 1 1/2 cups (360 ml) dairy-free milk of choice
- Whole pecans to decorate

Instructions

1. Preheat the oven to 375 °F (190 °C).
2. Add all dry ingredients to a baking dish and stir with a spoon.
3. Add the wet ingredients and stir to combine.

4. Transfer the dish to the oven and bake for 35 minutes, or until the edges are golden, and the center has set.
5. Finally, allow the pumpkin oatmeal bake to cool and optionally frost it with cashew cream, and decorate with whole pecans. Enjoy!

Prep Time: 15 Minutes

Cook Time: 25 Minutes

Servings: 5

Ingredients

- 1 tbsp oil
- 1 medium white onion diced
- 3 medium (200 g) carrots diced
- 5 small (500 g) potatoes chopped
- 1 medium (70 g) stalk celery with greens, finely sliced
- 3 garlic cloves minced
- 1/2 to 1 tbsp fresh thyme or 1 tsp dried
- 1/2 to 1 tbsp fresh rosemary or 1 tsp dried
- 1/2 to 1 tbsp fresh oregano or 1 tsp dried
- 1 1/2 tsp sea salt or to taste
- 1/2 tsp black pepper or to taste
- 1/3 tsp nutmeg
- 1/4 tsp smoked paprika
- 1/4 tsp red pepper flakes or less if sensitive to heat
- 3 cups (720 ml) low-sodium vegetable broth or water
- 2 1/3 cup (350 g) frozen peas
- 1/2 cup (120 g) dairy-free heavy cream or canned coconut milk
- 2 tbsp cornstarch or arrowroot flour
- 1/2 cup (120 ml) white wine or more vegetable broth

Instructions

1. Heat oil over medium heat in a pan and add the onion. Sauté for about 2-4 minutes, stirring frequently.
2. Add carrots, potatoes, celery, garlic, and all herbs + spices. Sauté for a further one minute, then add vegetable broth.
3. Bring to a boil over high heat. Cook for about 5 minutes over low-medium heat, then add the frozen peas and cook for 15 more minutes, or until the veggies and peas are softened, stirring occasionally.
4. In a small bowl, mix cornstarch with vegan heavy cream or canned coconut milk with a whisk.
5. Pour the milk into the stew, also add white wine (or use more broth/or plant-based milk for a creamier soup) and let simmer for a further 3-4 minutes.
6. Taste and adjust seasonings. Add more salt/pepper/spices to taste. You can blend half of the soup with an immersion blender to make it creamier.
7. Garnish with fresh herbs (optional) and enjoy! Store leftovers covered in the refrigerator for up to 3 days. The stew can be frozen!

Prep Time: 5 Minutes

Cook Time: 00 Minutes

Servings: 10

Ingredients

- 1 cup (150 g) cashews
- 1/2 cup (120 ml) water or dairy-free milk
- Salt to taste (optional)
- Lemon juice to taste (optional)

Instructions

1. First, leave the cashews to soak overnight in the fridge in a bowl filled with plenty of cold water. If you're running low on time, you could boil them for 15 minutes until softened (then drain).
2. Transfer the cashews and fresh water to a high-speed blender and process until smooth and creamy (see further water ratios below in the notes). Pause to scrape down the sides of the blender as needed to ensure it's thoroughly blended.
3. Transfer the blended cream to an airtight container and store it in the fridge for up to 4 days. Enjoy!

Prep Time: 10 Minutes

Cook Time: 20 Minutes

Servings: 6

Ingredients

- 1 1/2 cups (300 g) dry red lentils
- 1 large (200 g) carrot finely diced
- 1 small bell pepper
- 1 large onion chopped
- 4 cloves of garlic minced
- 1 heaped tbsp fresh ginger minced
- 1/2 tbsp vegetable oil
- 3 cups (720 ml) vegetable broth or water
- 1 cup (240 ml) canned coconut milk
- 1 1/2 tsp ground cumin
- 1 tbsp curry powder
- 1/2 tbsp sweetener of choice
- 1 tsp ground turmeric
- 1 tsp paprika
- Sea salt and black pepper to taste
- 1/3 tsp red pepper flakes (optional)

Instructions

1. Rinse lentils under running water. Chop the onion, garlic, ginger, bell pepper, and carrot.

2. Heat oil in a pot and sauté onion for about 3-4 minutes over medium heat. Add ginger, garlic, carrot, and bell pepper.
3. Add all spices, sweetener, lentils, and vegetable broth or water. Bring to a boil and let simmer for about 10 minutes.
4. Finally, add coconut milk and cook for a further 5 minutes or until the desired thickness of the dhal is reached.
5. Season with black pepper and salt. Taste and adjust the seasonings as needed.
6. Serve warm with basmati rice, potatoes, or naan (flatbread) and garnish with fresh herbs.

Prep Time: 15 Minutes

Cook Time: 20 Minutes

Servings: 10

Ingredients

Buffalo chickpea sauce:

- 1 tbsp vegetable oil
- 1 medium-sized onion chopped
- 2 cloves of garlic minced
- 1 bell pepper chopped
- 1 1/2 cups cooked chickpeas (or one 15 Oz can, drained and rinsed)
- 1/2 cup tomato sauce (passata)
- 3 tbsp hot sauce (or more to taste)
- 2 tbsp plant-based milk
- 1 tbsp balsamic vinegar
- 1 tsp onion powder
- 3/4 tsp coconut sugar (or brown sugar)
- 1/2 tsp garlic powder
- 1/2 tsp smoked paprika
- 1/2 tsp ground cumin

Sea salt & black pepper to taste

Chili powder to taste

Tortillas:

- 10 small flour tortillas (gluten-free if needed) about 14 cm in diameter

- Dipping Sauce (optional):
- Vegan cheese sauce (or your favorite dipping sauce)

Instructions

1. Using a fork, roughly mash the chickpeas in a bowl.
2. Heat oil in a pan/skillet over medium heat and add the chopped onion and bell pepper. Cook for 3 minutes, then add garlic and spice mix and sauté for a further minute.
3. Add all other sauce ingredients + chickpeas to the pan and bring the mixture to a boil. Let simmer on low heat for about 2-4 minutes, stirring occasionally, then turn off the heat.
4. Taste the mixture, if you want it spicier, add more chili powder to taste.
5. Preheat oven to 410 degrees F (210 degrees C) and line a baking sheet with parchment paper.
6. Place about 2 tbsp of the filling onto each tortilla and roll them up tightly. Place every tortilla seam-side down on the baking sheet, next to each other.
7. Brush them with a little bit of vegetable oil (to make them even more crispy).
8. Bake in the oven for about 15-20 minutes or until they are golden brown and crispy.
9. Drizzle with vegan cheese sauce (optional) or top them with your favorite vegan cheese before baking. Enjoy with your favorite dip!

11. Vegan Yum Yum Sauce

Prep Time: 5 Minutes

Cook Time: 00 Minutes

Servings: 10

Ingredients

- 1 cup (240 g) vegan sour cream or vegan mayonnaise
- 1 1/2 tbsp tomato paste or ketchup
- 1/2 tbsp maple syrup
- 2 tsp rice vinegar
- 1 tsp garlic powder
- 1 tsp onion powder
- 1/2 tsp smoked paprika
- 1 pinch of Kala Nampak if using sour cream
- Salt to taste
- Water too thin to desired consistency

Instructions

1. Add all ingredients to a small-medium bowl and stir with a whisk until combined. Start with 1 tbsp of water and add more if you want a runnier sauce.
2. Taste it and adjust seasonings as needed. I also like to add a little hot sauce for some heat.
3. Cover the bowl and chill for a few hours (or overnight) which will help the flavors to mend.
4. Store leftovers in an airtight container in the refrigerator for up to 6 days.

Prep Time: 10 Minutes

Cook Time: 25 Minutes

Servings: 4

Ingredients

Roasted veggies:

- 1 cup (180 g) cherry tomatoes
- 1 sweet pepper sliced (color of choice)
- 1 small head of garlic
- 1 1/2 tbsp olive oil
- 2 pinches of sea salt

White Bean Dip:

- 1 1/2 cups white beans canned, drained and rinsed
- 1/3 tsp sea salt
- 1/2 tsp onion powder
- 2 tsp nutritional yeast
- 1/2 tsp Italian seasoning

Black pepper to taste:

- 1 1/2 tbsp (24 g) tahini or cashew butter
- 1 1/2 tbsp lemon juice
- 6-8 tbsp water to thin
- Parsley for garnish (optional)

Instructions

1. Preheat the oven to 400 °F (205 °C), then cut off the top of the head of garlic (about 1/4-1/2 inch resp. 0, 6-1, 2 cm).
2. Add the cherry tomatoes, pepper, and garlic to a baking dish and drizzle with oil, and season with salt. Cover the garlic with a ramekin (or use tin foil) and roast for about 30 minutes.
3. Let the garlic cool until you can handle it, then gently squeeze the garlic cloves from the head until they pop out into the blender. Also, add all other dip ingredients (but not the roasted veggies) and blend until completely smooth. Use enough water to blend, start with a few tablespoons, and then increase as needed.
4. Transfer the mixture to a shallow bowl, and create a swirl with the back of a spoon.
5. Top with the roasted tomatoes and sliced pepper (along with the remaining oil from the baking dish) and sprinkle with fresh parsley and optionally chili powder. Enjoy with naan or pita.

Prep Time: 10 Minutes

Cook Time: 20 Minutes

Servings: 8

Ingredients

- One 15 oz can (280 g) chickpeas (rinsed and drained)
- 1 medium-sized onion
- 2 cloves garlic
- Juice of 1/2 lime
- 1 tsp onion powder
- 1 tsp ground cumin
- 1/2 tsp ground oregano
- 1/2 tsp smoked paprika
- 1/4 tsp red pepper flakes
- Sea salt & pepper to taste
- 1/3 cup (50 g) rice flour
- 1 cup fresh (160 g) corn (or canned)
- 1 bell pepper chopped
- 2 tbsp parsley chopped
- Vegetable oil for frying
- Vegan cheese (optional)
- Cashew dip (optional)

Instructions

1. Watch the video to see all the instruction steps.
2. Process chickpeas, onion, garlic, lime juice, and all spices in a food processor.

3. Add rice flour and mix again.
4. Put the mixture into a bowl and add the chopped pepper, corn, and parsley. Stir with a spoon or use your hands.
5. Form 8 patties and fry them with some oil in a skillet from both sides (about 5 minutes each) until golden brown.
6. Serve with a cashew dip. Enjoy!

Prep Time: 10 Minutes

Cook Time: 15 Minutes

Servings: 12

Ingredients

Tofu & Veggies:

- 8 oz (225 g) firm tofu
- 2 tomatoes
- 8-12 mushrooms
- 1 green pepper
- 1/2 zucchini
- 1 cup pineapple cubed (optional)

Marinade:

- 1 1/2 tbsp maple syrup
- 2 1/2 tbsp soy sauce
- 2 tbsp (32 g) peanut butter melted
- 1 tbsp oil
- 2 tbsp BBQ Sauce
- 1 tsp hot sauce
- 1 tsp onion powder
- 1 tsp garlic powder
- Black pepper to taste
- 3 tbsp water

Other ingredients

Peanut sauce to serve

- 8-12 wood or bamboo skewers soak in water (see instructions)

Instructions

Ofu & Veggies:

1. Place the tofu between a kitchen towels and place a heavy pan on top. Press for about 30 minutes. You can cut the tofu into cubes before pressing or after.
2. Cut the veggies into a similar size.
3. Marinade
4. Add all marinade ingredients (except the water) to a bowl and mix thoroughly with a whisk. Add the water in 3 portions, mixing in between. Set aside.
5. Assemble
6. Transfer the veggies and tofu to a shallow dish and add the marinade. Carefully stir with a spatula to cover the veggies/tofu with the marinade from all sides.
7. Marinate in the refrigerator for about 60 minutes (or overnight if preparing the recipe one day in advance). At the same time soak wood or bamboo skewers in water for 30-60 minutes.
8. Drain the marinade into a bowl (don't throw it away) and thread the veggies and cubes of tofu onto skewers.
9. Cook in a pan
10. Heat a grill pan, brush it with a little oil (using a silicone brush) and place the skewers in. Cook for about 4-5 minutes on each side (brushing with the marinade in between) until the vegetables start getting a light char and the tofu turns golden brown.
11. Remove from the pan and serve with peanut sauce, sprinkle with sesame seeds and fresh herbs. Enjoy!
12. Bake

13. Preheat the oven to 390 F (200 C) and place the skewers in a baking dish.
14. Pour the remaining marinade over the skewers and bake for about 25 minutes, flipping once after 15 minutes.
15. Remove from the oven and serve with peanut sauce, sprinkle with sesame seeds and fresh herbs. Enjoy!

Prep Time: 20 Minutes

Cook Time: 25 Minutes

Servings: 10

Ingredients

Dough:

- 2 cups (205 g) oats gluten-free if needed
- 1 cup (120 g) almond flour
- 1 cup (90 g) oat flour (ground oats) gluten-free if needed
- 1 small (80 g) banana mashed
- 1/4 cup (80 g) maple syrup or agave syrup
- 1/4 cup (60 g) coconut milk canned
- 2 tsp baking powder

Strawberry Filling:

- 3 cups (450 g) diced strawberries
- 1/3 cup (105 g) maple syrup or agave syrup
- 2-3 tsp lime or lemon juice
- 5 tsp chia seeds
- 3 tsp potato starch or cornstarch

Instructions

1. I recommend using a kitchen scale for this recipe and measuring the ingredients in grams. The recipe has a video for visual instructions.

2. Preheat the oven to 360 degrees Fahrenheit (180 degrees Celsius).
3. Put the ingredients for the strawberry filling in a saucepan, bring to a boil, let it simmer for 5-10 minutes, and stir occasionally.
4. Mix all ingredients for the dough in a bowl by either using your hands or a hand mixer.
5. Press 2/3 of the dough evenly into a greased or lined baking dish. My pan measures 7 x 11 inches (18 x 28 cm).
6. Pour the strawberry filling over the crust.
7. Crumble the remaining 1/3 dough on top.
8. Bake in the oven for 20-25 minutes. Enjoy!

Prep Time: 15 Minutes

Cook Time: 25 Minutes

Servings: 8

Ingredients

Dry ingredients:

- 1 heaped cup (100 g) oat flour (gluten-free if needed
- 1 cup (140 g) gluten-free flour blend or regular flour
- 1 1/2 tsp baking powder
- 1/4 tsp baking soda
- 1/4 tsp salt

Wet ingredients:

- 3/4 cup (180 ml) plant-based milk of choice
- 1/3 cup (105 g) maple syrup
- 2 1/2 tbsp (30 g) oil
- 1 tbsp lemon juice or lime juice
- 1 1/2 tsp vanilla extract
- 1 1/2 cups (150 g) blueberries fresh or frozen

Instructions

1. I recommend measuring the ingredients in grams on a kitchen scale. Preheat oven to 360 degrees Fahrenheit (180 degrees Celsius) and line a muffin pan with paper liners or grease the pan.

2. Add plant-based milk and lemon juice to a small/medium bowl. Stir to combine and set aside for a few minutes to make "vegan buttermilk".
3. Meanwhile, add all dry ingredients to a large mixing bowl and stir with a whisk.
4. Now add the wet ingredients and stir with a spatula or whisk to combine. Do not over mix the batter. Finally, fold in the blueberries.
5. Divide the batter among the wells of the muffin pan. I had enough batter to make 8 muffins.
6. Bake for 25-30 minutes or until you spot cracks on top of the muffins. You can also make a toothpick test. Insert the toothpick into the center of a muffin. It should come out fairly clean (it's ok if the toothpick is crumbly but it shouldn't come out wet).
7. Let the muffins cool and enjoy! Store leftovers in an airtight container in the refrigerator for up to 5-6 days or freeze for up to 3 months. They won't stay soft if stored in the fridge, however, you can reheat them in the oven until warmed through to make them softer again.

Prep Time: 5 Minutes

Cook Time: 15 Minutes

Servings: 5

Ingredients

- 1 cup (90 g) oat flour (gluten-free if needed)
- 2/3 cup (160 ml) lite coconut milk (canned)
- 1/2 (65 g) banana
- Optional ingredients
- 1-2 tbsp maple syrup for sweeter pancakes
- 3/4 tsp baking powder for fluffier pancakes
- Pinch of salt

Instructions

1. I recommend measuring the ingredients in grams on a kitchen scale.
2. In a bowl, mash the banana with a fork, add the other ingredients and stir with a whisk until just combined.
3. Heat a little oil in a skillet over medium heat. Spoon some of the batter (I use one heaping ice cream scoop) into the hot skillet and cook the pancake on low to medium from both sides until golden brown.
4. Serve with either fruit, maple syrup, a chocolate sauce, caramel sauce, or whatever you prefer. Enjoy!

Prep Time: 15 Minutes

Cook Time: 40 Minutes

Servings: 8

Ingredients

Dry ingredients:

- 2 cups (200 g) oat flour (gluten-free if needed)
- 1/2 cup (100 g) granulated sweetener of choice
- 3/4 cup (75 g) almond flour (ground almonds)
- 1 1/2 tsp baking powder
- 1/4 tsp salt
- 1/3 cup (60 g) dairy-free chocolate chips + more for the top

Wet ingredients:

- 3/4 cup (180 ml) plant-based milk
- 2 medium (200 g) super ripe bananas
- 1/2 tbsp vinegar or lemon juice
- 1 tsp vanilla extract

Instructions

1. I recommend measuring the ingredients in grams on a kitchen scale.
2. Also, watch the video for easy visual instructions.
3. Preheat the oven to 360 degrees F (180 degrees C) and line an 8-inch baking pan with parchment paper.

4. Place all dry ingredients (except the chocolate chips) into a large bowl and mix with a whisk. You can also process the ingredients in a food processor (that's what I did).
5. In a small/medium bowl, mash the bananas really well (e.g. with a fork) and add them to the bowl (or food processor) with the dry ingredients.
6. Add the plant-based milk, vinegar, and vanilla extract and whisk again or use the pulse function of your food processor until just combined (don't over mix).
7. Finally, add the chocolate chips and stir with a spoon.
8. Pour the batter into the baking pan and add more chocolate chips on top.
9. Bake the bread in the oven for about 40 minutes (you don't want to over bake it). Check the center with a toothpick- if it comes out dry or slightly sticky/crumbly, that's fine, just not wet.
10. Let the banana bread cool, slice it, and enjoy!

Prep Time: 15 Minutes

Cook Time: 20 Minutes

Servings: 4

Ingredients

Creamy veggies:

- 1 tbsp vegan butter or oil
- ½ large onion chopped
- 3 garlic cloves finely minced
- 1 ½ cups of (215 g) carrots diced
- 1 ½ cups of (215 g) frozen peas thawed
- 2 cups (200 g) cauliflower chopped into small florets
- 1 ¼ cups of (180 g) corn fresh from the cob or from a jar/can
- 1 ½ cups (360 ml) plant-based cream/milk
- ½ cup (120 ml) vegetable broth
- 2 tbsp cornstarch or arrowroot flour or regular flour
- ½ tsp sea salt or to taste

Black pepper to taste

Red pepper flakes to taste:

- ½ tbsp fresh thyme or to taste
- 1 tbsp Dijon mustard
- 1 tbsp nutritional yeast (optional)
- ½ tbsp lemon juice

Mashed potatoes:

- 4 medium-sized (600 g) potatoes

- ¼ cup (60 ml) plant-based cream/milk
- ½ tsp nutmeg or to taste
- Sea salt to taste
- Black pepper to taste

Instructions

1. Sauté the onion with vegan butter (margarine) or some oil in a skillet/pan. After a few minutes, add garlic, cauliflower, and carrots. Pour in the vegetable broth and let it all simmer for a further 8-10 minutes with a closed lid at low heat.
2. In the meantime, peel the potatoes and cut them into pieces, then add them to a pot with boiling salted water. Cook the potatoes over medium heat for about 10-15 minutes or until they are fork-tender. Drain the potato water, then add the potatoes back into the pot. Add the plant-based cream/milk and the spices. Mash it all together with a potato masher, until it becomes a potato puree (don't use a food processor or a blender, otherwise the puree will turn out sticky).
3. After 8-10 minutes, add the thawed peas and the corn to the pan. Next, stir in the spices, mustard, and lemon juice.
4. Mix the plant-based cream and cornstarch in a bowl using a whisk. Pour this mixture into the pan and stir. It thickens up after a short time.
5. Taste and adjust seasonings. Feel free to add more salt, pepper, thyme, lemon juice or mustard. If the sauce is too thick, add a splash of plant-based cream/milk. If it's too thin, simply add more cornstarch or flour (mixed with plant-based milk or cream).

6. Serve and enjoy the creamed vegetables with mashed
    potatoes. Store leftovers in an airtight container for up
    to 3 days in the fridge or freeze for up to three month.

Prep Time: 20 Minutes

Cook Time: 28 Minutes

Servings: 3

Ingredients

Vegan meatballs:

- 1 (15 oz) can black beans drained and rinsed (250 g)
- 1/4 cup (35 g) sunflower seeds
- 1/2 cup (45 g) oats (gluten-free if needed)
- 2 tbsp (60 g) tomato paste
- 2 cloves of garlic
- 1/2 large onion chopped
- 2 tbsp ground chia seeds or flax seeds
- 1/2 tbsp onion powder
- 1 tsp garlic powder
- 1 tsp oregano
- 1 tsp ground cumin
- 1/2 tsp smoked paprika
- 1/4 tsp red pepper flakes (optional)
- Sea salt and pepper to taste
- Oil for frying

Gravy:

- 1 1/2 cups (360 ml) vegetable broth or water
- 1/3 cup (80 ml) plant-based cream or canned coconut milk
- 2 tbsp (60 g) tomato paste
- 1/2 tsp fresh ginger (minced)

- 3 tsp curry powder
- 1 1/2 tsp onion powder
- 1 tsp garlic powder
- 1 tsp oregano
- 1 tsp cumin
- 1 tsp turmeric (optional)
- 1/2 tsp nutmeg
- 1/2 tsp smoked paprika
- 1/4 tsp red pepper flakes (optional)
- 1 tsp coconut sugar (or brown sugar)
- Sea salt and pepper to taste
- 1 tbsp cornstarch (to thicken)
- Fresh parsley to garnish

Instructions

1. Prepare mashed potatoes or make your favorite pasta or rice (whatever you want to serve with your vegan meatballs).
2. Vegan meatballs:
3. Put all the meatball ingredients (except oil) into a food processor (or blender) and pulse a couple of times. Scrape down the sides and pulse again. Repeat for about one minute or until the mixture sticks together in a thick paste.
4. Roll the mixture with your hands into balls. I used 1 tbsp per ball (the recipe makes about 15 balls).
5. Preheat oven to 390 degrees F (200 degrees C).
6. Heat 2-3 tbsp oil in a pan/skillet and fry the balls for about 6-8 minutes over medium heat. Shake the pan from time to time to fry the balls evenly on all sides.

7. Transfer the balls onto a baking sheet and bake for about 20 minutes.

Gravy:

1. To make the gravy, add the tomato paste to a pan (use the same pan which you used for the meatless balls), pour in the plant-based cream, and stir with a whisk to smooth out the tomato paste. Then slowly add the vegetable broth, while stirring.
2. Bring the sauce to a boil, add all other ingredients (except cornstarch and fresh parsley) and allow it to simmer over medium heat for 10-12 minutes (the longer you simmer the gravy, the more flavorful and thicker it will be).
3. In a small bowl mix cornstarch with a little bit of water into a 'slurry' and then add it to the pan. The gravy will get a little bit thicker. Keep simmering for a further 2-3 minutes.
4. Pour the gravy over the meat-free balls and serve with either mashed potatoes, pasta, or rice! Store leftovers of the gravy and meatballs (separated) in the fridge for 3-4 days.

21. One-Pot Pasta

Prep Time: 8 Minutes

Cook Time: 12 Minutes

Servings: 3

Ingredients

- 8 oz (225 g) dry pasta gluten-free or regular
- 1/2 tbsp veggie bouillon powder
- 1 tsp onion powder
- 1 tsp garlic powder
- 1 tsp salt
- 1/2 tsp black pepper
- 1/2 tsp paprika
- 3 garlic cloves minced
- 1 small/medium (120 g) onion red or yellow, chopped
- 1 2/3 cup (120 g) broccoli florets
- 1 cup (125 g) zucchini chopped
- 1 cup (85 g) red pepper chopped
- 2 cups (480 ml) water
- 1 1/4 cup (300 g) passata
- 1/2 cup (120 g) canned coconut milk

Instructions

1. Add all ingredients to a large pot (or skillet with deep sides) and stir to combine. Bring it to a boil over high heat.

2. Once it starts boiling, reduce the heat to low and set the timer to 12 minutes. Cook until the pasta is al-dente, stirring every few minutes.
3. Depending on the type and shape of the pasta, the cooking time will vary. that gluten-free noodles/ pasta usually takes less time, and larger/thicker pasta varieties may take longer.
4. Serve in bowls, garnish with fresh herbs like parsley, and enjoy!

Prep Time: 15 Minutes

Cook Time: 30 Minutes

Servings: 4

Ingredients

- 1 tbsp oil
- 1 onion chopped
- 1 celery stalk diced
- 1 bell pepper chopped
- 5 oz (140 g) mushrooms sliced (optional)
- 2 garlic cloves minced
- 1 tsp dried oregano
- 1 tsp onion powder
- 1 tsp brown sugar
- 3/4 tsp ground cumin
- 3/4 tsp turmeric powder
- 1/2 tsp ground coriander
- 1/2 tsp smoked paprika powder
- 1/4 tsp red pepper flakes or to taste
- Sea salt & pepper to taste
- 1 cup dry lentils (I used brown)
- 3 cups of vegetable broth
- 2 dried bay leaves
- 14 oz (400 g) crushed tomatoes
- 1 1/2 cups (150 g) okra chopped
- 15 oz can of (250 g) cannellini beans or cooked beans of choice
- 1 tbsp balsamic vinegar

- 2 tbsp soy sauce (gluten-free if needed)
- 1 tsp cornstarch mixed with 1-2 tbsp plant-based milk to thicken (optional)
- Fresh herbs e.g. parsley to garnish

Instructions

1. Heat oil in a pot over medium heat and add the chopped onion, celery, bell pepper, and mushrooms. Cook for 5 minutes, then add garlic and cook for 2 more minutes.
2. Add the spices, the lentils, and broth and bring the mixture to a boil.
3. Now add the bay leaves and cook the vegan Gumbo with a lid on for about 15 minutes.
4. Then add the crushed tomatoes and okra and stir. Let the Gumbo simmer for a further 10-15 minutes or until the lentils are cooked but not mushy.
5. Finally, add the soy sauce, balsamic vinegar, and the cooked beans.
6. You can also mix 1 tsp of cornstarch with 1-2 tbsp plant-based milk and add it to the Gumbo to thicken.
7. Taste it, if you want it spicier, add more red pepper flakes, or hot sauce to taste.
8. Garnish with fresh herbs and enjoy! Can be served with rice, potatoes or bread.

Prep Time: 10 Minutes

Cook Time: 20 Minutes

Servings: 2

Ingredients

- 1 onion diced
- 2-3 garlic cloves minced
- 1 tbsp vegetable oil
- 11 oz (300 g) fresh mushrooms sliced
- 4 tbsp (40 ml) white wine (optional)
- 1 tbsp tamari or soy sauce
- 3/4 cup (180 ml) vegetable broth or water
- 3/4 cup (180 ml) plant-based milk or cream
- 2 tbsp cornstarch
- 1 tsp onion powder
- 1/2 tsp garlic powder
- 1/2 tsp smoked paprika
- A pinch of red pepper flakes
- Salt & black pepper to taste
- 1 tbsp nutritional yeast flakes (optional)
- Fresh thyme leaves and/or parsley (and/or tarragon) chopped
- Serve with rice or pasta of choice

Instructions

1. Heat oil in a large pan/skillet, add onion and fry for about 5 minutes. Add garlic and fry for a further 1 minute.
2. Now add the mushrooms and fry over medium heat for about 5 minutes.
3. Pour in white wine (optional), vegetable broth, tamari (or soy sauce), and the spice mixture. I love adding nutritional yeast flakes as well but that's optional! Bring to a boil.
4. Add cornstarch to the plant-based milk or cream (I used canned coconut milk, however, almond milk, oat milk/cream or soy milk/cream is fine too) and stir to dissolve.
5. Pour the milk/cream mixture into the pan and cook on low-medium heat for about 10 minutes until the sauce thickens. Taste and adjust seasonings as to your preference.
6. Add fresh thyme leaves and/or parsley and/or tarragon to taste! Enjoy with brown rice or pasta of choice! This creamy mushroom sauce also tastes great over mashed potatoes!

Prep Time: 15 Minutes

Cook Time: 30 Minutes

Servings: 8

Ingredients

Dough:

- 1 kg (2 pounds) potatoes
- 80 g (1/2 cup) white rice flour
- 40 g (1/3 cup) cornstarch or tapioca flour (1/3 cup)
- Salt, pepper, nutmeg (to taste)

Filling:

- 250 g (3 cups) mushrooms sliced
- 1/2 of a zucchini diced
- 1 onion chopped
- 1 bell pepper diced
- 2 cloves of garlic minced
- Salt & pepper to taste
- 1 tsp Italian spice blend
- 1 tsp onion powder
- 1 tsp garlic powder
- 1/2 tsp cumin
- 1/4 tsp red pepper flakes
- Additional ingredients:
- Oil for frying
- Vegan cheese to taste (optional)

Instructions

Dough:

1. Peel potatoes, cut into small pieces, and cook in salted water for about 20 minutes.
2. Season with salt, pepper, and nutmeg and mash them with a potato masher. (Please do not use a food processor, otherwise, the mashed potatoes will be sticky).
3. Allow the mashed potatoes to cool (in the meantime you can prepare the filling), then add flour and cornstarch and mix well with a spoon or your hands.

Filling:

1. Chop the veggies into small pieces, fry the onion in a pan with a little oil for about 3-4 minutes, add the mushrooms, garlic, and also the diced peppers and the zucchini. Sauté everything for a couple of minutes, season with salt, pepper, and the spice mix.
2. Split the dough into 8 parts (about 1/2 cup or 120 g each). Form into balls, make a well in the middle, and add about one and a half tablespoons of the filling. You can also add some vegan cheese (I used vegan cheese sauce) in addition. Carefully "seal" the balls with more dough and flatten them slightly to make them look like thick pancakes.
3. Heat approximately 2 tablespoons of oil in a pan and fry the potato cakes at medium heat until golden brown on both sides. They will be crunchy on the outside and soft on the inside. If you want them to be slightly more crunchy, you can bake them additionally for about 20 minutes at 375 degrees Fahrenheit in the oven. Enjoy!

Prep Time: 15 Minutes

Cook Time: 35 Minutes

Servings: 3

Ingredients

Mushroom Bourguignon:

- 1 oz (28 g) dried mushrooms OR 10 oz fresh sliced mushrooms
- 1 tbsp oil
- 1/2 large onion diced
- 2 small/medium (140 g) carrots chopped
- 2/3 cup (100 g) peas frozen (optional)
- 3 garlic cloves minced
- 3/4 tbsp fresh thyme or 1 tsp dried thyme
- 1 tsp onion powder
- 3/4 tsp sea salt or to taste
- 1/4 tsp black pepper or to taste
- 1/4 tsp smoked paprika
- 1/3 cup (80 ml) red wine
- 1/2 tbsp tamari or soy sauce
- 3/4 cup (180 ml) vegetable broth + 1/4 cup more if needed
- 1/4 cup (60 ml) plant-based milk
- 3/4 tbsp cornstarch or arrowroot flour
- Mashed Potatoes:
- 4 medium-sized (600 g) potatoes
- 1/4 cup (60 ml) coconut milk canned
- 1/2 tsp nutmeg or to taste

- Black pepper & sea salt to taste

Instructions

1. Soak dried mushrooms in warm water for about 15-20 minutes, then drain. Skip this step if you are using fresh mushrooms.
2. Meanwhile, peel and chop potatoes, add them to a pot with water and salt. Bring to a boil. Cook on medium heat for about 15 minutes or until tender, drain. Transfer back to the pot, add coconut milk, nutmeg, black pepper, and sea salt to taste and mash with a potato masher (don't use a food processor or blender). Set aside.
3. Heat oil in a pan over medium heat. Add onion and sauté for 4-5 minutes. Add drained mushrooms, carrot, peas, garlic, thyme, and all spices. Sauté for a further one minute, stirring frequently.
4. Add red wine. Cook for about 2 minutes. Then add tamari (or soy sauce), and vegetable broth.
5. Let simmer over low/medium heat with a lid on for about 10-12 minutes or until the carrots and peas are softened.
6. Combine plant-based milk and cornstarch in a bowl, stir with a whisk until there are no lumps. Add the mixture to the pan and stir (the sauce will thicken). Let simmer for a few more minutes.
7. Taste and adjust seasonings. Add more salt/pepper/spices if needed. Serve mushroom bourguignon with mashed potatoes and enjoy! Store leftovers covered in the refrigerator for up to 3 days.

Prep Time: 15 Minutes

Cook Time: 25 Minutes

Servings: 4

Ingredients

- 1 tbsp oil
- 1 medium onion finely diced
- 1 medium (52 g) stalk celery finely diced (1/2 cup)
- 10 oz fresh (280 g) mushrooms finely diced (or 1 oz dried)
- 2 medium (200 g) carrots finely grated
- 4 cloves garlic finely minced or crushed
- 2 tsp Italian seasoning or use 1 tsp each of dried oregano and basil
- 1 tsp onion powder
- 1 tsp coconut sugar or sweetener of choice
- Pinch of red pepper flakes or to taste
- Salt and black pepper to taste
- 1/3 cup (80 ml) red wine or use more vegetable broth
- 3 cups (750 g) crushed tomatoes or marinara sauce or tomato sauce
- 2 cups (480 ml) vegetable broth
- 1 bay leaf
- 1 cup (200 g) dry lentils I used brown, soaked
- 1 tbsp soy sauce gluten-free if needed or tamari
- 1 tbsp balsamic vinegar
- 1/2 cup (120 ml) plant-based milk
- 1 tsp cornstarch

- 8 oz (225 g) spaghetti gluten-free if needed or pasta of choice
- Vegan parmesan or nutritional yeast to garnish (optional)

Instructions

1. I recommend soaking the lentils in lukewarm water if you are using green or brown lentils. This step is optional, however, the lentils cook faster and are furthermore better digested when soaked. You can skip this step if using red lentils.
2. Heat oil in a pan or pot over medium heat. Add onion, celery, mushrooms, and carrots. Sauté for 3-4 minutes. Stir in garlic, sweetener,and all spices. Sauté for a further one minute, stirring frequently.
3. Add red wine (or vegetable broth), crushed tomatoes, vegetable broth, the bay leaf, and the drained lentils. Stir to combine.
4. Bring to a boil and let simmer for 20 minutes or until the lentils are tender (depending on the variety it can take shorter or longer).
5. Meanwhile, cook your favorite pasta (e.g. spaghetti) as per package instructions.
6. Add soy sauce and balsamic vinegar. Mix the plant-based milk and cornstarch in a small bowl and add the mixture to the pan.
7. Taste and adjust seasonings. Add more salt/pepper/spices to taste. Also, add more vegetable broth if needed.
8. Serve the lentil bolognese in bowls over pasta and sprinkle vegan Parmesan on top (optional). Enjoy!

Store bolognese sauce leftovers covered in the refrigerator for up to 4 days.

Prep Time: 10 Minutes

Cook Time: 20 Minutes

Servings: 5

Ingredients

- 1/2 tbsp oil
- 2 medium (320 g) potatoes diced
- 1 medium (120 g) carrot chopped
- 2 (60 g) celery stalks with greens, chopped
- 3 garlic cloves minced
- 1 1/2 tsp onion powder
- 3/4 tsp dried oregano
- 1/2 tsp dried marjoram
- 1/3 tsp red pepper flakes
- 4-5 cups (1100 ml) vegetable broth or water
- 2 bay leaves (optional)
- Salt & pepper to taste
- Three 14 oz cans white beans (about 4 cups), rinsed and drained
- 1/4 cup (60 ml) coconut milk canned
- 1/2 to 1 cup kale chopped (optional)
- Fresh herbs to garnish

Instructions

1. Chop the potatoes, celery, and carrot and mince the garlic.

2. Heat oil in a large pot over medium heat and add the garlic, all veggies, potatoes, and spices (onion powder, oregano, marjoram, red pepper flakes, salt, and pepper). Saute for about one minute.
3. Pour in the vegetable broth (or water) and bring the soup to a boil. Add the bay leaves (optional).
4. Let the soup simmer for about 10 minutes, then add the white beans and coconut milk. Simmer for a further 5-10 minutes.
5. Pour a part of the soup (e.g. half of it) to a different pot. Take out the bay leaves (if you used them).
6. Blend this part using an immersion blender until its smooth. You can also blend the soup in a regular blender. Make sure to work in batches and not to overfill the blender.
7. Pour the blended soup back to the large pot and stir to combine. If you want to have an even thicker soup/chowder, you can blend all the soup.
8. Taste and adjust seasoning. Add more salt/pepper to taste and red pepper flakes to add more heat.
9. Garnish with fresh herbs (e.g. parsley), and enjoy. Serve with bread or toast.

Prep Time: 20 Minutes

Cook Time: 40 Minutes

Servings: 8

Ingredients

- 2 large (400 g) potatoes peeled, or sweet potato
- 1 tbsp oil
- 2/3 cup (100 g) onion chopped
- 2 medium-sized (100 g) celery stalks chopped
- 3 garlic cloves minced
- 1/2 tbsp onion powder
- 3/4 tsp sea salt
- 1/2 tsp caraway seeds
- 1/2 tsp ground cumin
- 1/2 tsp dried thyme
- 1/2 tsp smoked paprika
- 1/3 tsp red pepper flakes
- Black pepper to taste
- 1 tbsp soy sauce tamari, or coconut amino
- 1 tbsp balsamic vinegar
- 2 (15 oz) cans black beans or kidney beans, about 500 g when drained and rinsed
- 1/2 cup (60 g) walnuts chopped or sunflower seeds for a nut-free version
- 1 cup (90 g) oats preferably instant oats
- 2 tbsp (60 g) tomato paste

Instructions

1. Chop the potatoes, transfer them to a pot with salted water and bring to a boil. Cook over medium heat for about 15 minutes or until tender, then drain. Transfer back to the pot and mash with a potato masher (don't use a food processor or blender).
2. Time to preheat the oven to 375 degrees F (190 degrees C).
3. Meanwhile, heat 1 tbsp oil in a skillet or pan over medium heat and add chopped onion. Fry for about 3 minutes, then add garlic, celery, all spices, soy sauce, and balsamic vinegar and fry for a further 3-5 minutes. Stir occasionally. Add beans and turn off the heat after one minute.
4. Transfer the bean/veggie mixture to the pot with the mashed potatoes and add tomato paste, oats, and chopped walnuts. Then, Use the potato masher or your hands to mix everything together.
5. Line an 8-inch or 9-inch loaf pan with parchment paper (including an overhang) and put the meatloaf mixture into the pan. Press it down firmly.
6. Bake the vegan loaf for 40-50 minutes, then remove from the oven and allow to rest for at least 15 minutes before removing it from the pan to avoid it breaking apart at all.
7. This meatless meatloaf needs time to firm up. When you first remove it from the pan, it will still be soft to the touch. Simply pop this in the fridge for at least three hours (or even overnight) before serving for the firmest results. Read the recipe notes for more ways to ensure a firmer loaf.

8. Serve with the mushroom sauce, maple tomato glaze,
    or gravy. I have included the recipe for the mushroom
    sauce and glaze below in the recipe notes.

Prep Time: 1 Minutes

Cook Time: 2 Minutes

Servings: 3

Ingredients

- 3/4 cup (180 ml) coconut milk canned
- 3 tbsp (20 g) nutritional yeast flakes
- 2 tbsp (15 g) tapioca flour OR arrowroot flour/starch
- 1/2 tsp sea salt (or to taste)
- 1/2 tsp onion powder (optional)
- 1/4 tsp garlic powder (optional)
- Pinch of smoked paprika (optional)

Instructions

1. Put all ingredients into a saucepan and stir with a whisk. Once everything is combined, turn on the heat and bring the mixture to a boil while stirring constantly.
2. Let simmer on low to medium heat for about one minute until the sauce is stretchy.
3. Enjoy this vegan cheese sauce with nachos, on pizza, over pasta, and many other savory dishes! Please read the recipe notes below.

Prep Time: 15 Minutes

Cook Time: 30 Minutes

Servings: 4

Ingredients

- 1 medium onion chopped
- 4 cloves of garlic finely minced
- 1 green pepper chopped
- 1 medium carrot grated
- 5-6 medium (560 g) diced fresh tomatoes or use 1 (20 oz) can
- 5 tbsp tomato paste
- 2 cups (480 ml) water or vegetable broth
- 4 cups cooked beans e.g. kidney beans, black beans, pinto beans, white beans, or 1 cup of each
- 2 tsp coconut sugar or sub brown sugar or any other sweetener like maple syrup
- 1 tsp ground cumin
- 1 tsp onion powder
- 1 tsp garlic powder
- 3/4 tsp salt or less if you use vegetable broth
- 1/2 tsp black pepper
- 1/4 tsp smoked paprika
- 1/4 tsp cayenne pepper
- 1-2 hot red chili peppers (I used 1, my partner prefers 2)
- 2 tsp oil of choice for frying

Instructions

1. In a large pan or pot over medium heat, add in the oil. Sauté the onion and pepper for about 5 minutes, add the garlic and sauté for an additional 1-2 minutes, stirring occasionally.
2. Mix in the tomatoes and sauté for another 3 to 5 minutes.
3. Now add all remaining ingredients, increase the heat and simmer for about 30 minutes or longer, stirring occasionally. Add more water or vegetable broth if the chili gets too thick.
4. Recommended step: Pour about 1 to 1 1/2 cups of the chili into a different pot. Blend this part using an immersion blender until smooth. You can also blend it in a regular blender. Pour the blended chili back into the large pot and stir to combine,
5. Serve with rice, pasta, potatoes or flatbread. Garnish with fresh cilantro or parsley.